When shopping at the grocery store, the foods you grab can greatly impact your overall health. In fact, filling your cart with a lot of refined grains, sugary drinks, and processed foods can increase inflammation and affect your health.

Therefore, filling up on healthy foods can help keep you healthy, protect against chronic diseases resistant to drugs and rid your body of toxins.

We also absorb tons of toxins every day through the air we breathe, the water we drink, the food we eat, and by just being outside in our surroundings.

So how do we get rid of these toxins that can be harmful to our body? It's through the Healing diet.

The Healing foods diet is not just a diet; It is a tool that will lead you to a total transformation of your health. This diet was designed to help everyone overcome diseases. It is designed to heal your body and improve your health by encouraging the consumption of nutritious, whole foods like fruits, veggies, legumes, healthy fats, organic meats, and healing herbs and spices.

Plus, this simple eating pattern is a great way to ensure you supply your body with a steady stream of the nutrients you need to help prevent nutritional deficiencies in your diet and to promote healthy living.

So what makes this diet unique?

This diet is unique because it involves making some simple switches in your diet compared to other complicated diets with many rules and regulations.

THE HEALING NEUROPATHY DIET RECIPES

1. Warm Wild Berry Smothered Sweet Potato

Prep: 30 mins

Cook: 1 hr 20 mins

Total: 1 hr 50 mins

Servings: 1

Ingredients

- 1 large sweet potato, cleaned
- ½ cup wild blueberries
- 2 tablespoon raw or roasted pecan pieces
- 1 teaspoon all-natural maple syrup (plus more for drizzling)
- ¼ teaspoon cinnamon
- ¼ teaspoon nutmeg
- ¼ teaspoon allspice
- ¼ teaspoon vanilla extract
- Pinch of sea salt

Directions

1. Preheat oven to 375 degrees.
2. Poke holes in potato, wrap in foil.
3. Bake 45-60 minutes. You will know it's done if a knife slides easily into the center.
4. When the potato is nearly done, toast pecans in dry saucepan (if desired), and warm berries.
5. When the potato is done, slice open top and scoop out flesh into a small bowl. Add spices, vanilla, sea salt and maple syrup to your liking and mix.
6. Fill potato shell with mixture.
7. Top potato with wild blueberries, sprinkle with pecans, and drizzle maple syrup, if desired.

Prep: 10 mins

Cook: 15 mins

Total: 25 mins

Servings: 4

Ingredients

- 4 cups frozen cooked brown rice
- 1-inch piece ginger
- 1/4 cup low-sodium soy sauce
- 1 to 2 tablespoons garlic chili sauce
- 1 tablespoon toasted sesame oil
- 12 ounces baked tofu
- 3 tablespoons canola oil
- One 3.5-ounce package sliced shiitake mushrooms (about 2 cups)
- One 1-pound package fresh stir-fry vegetable mix (not frozen)
- Kosher salt

- 1/2 cup roasted and salted cashew halves and pieces

Directions

1. Prepare the rice according to the package directions. Peel and finely grate the ginger and put it into a small baking dish or medium bowl along with the soy sauce, garlic chili sauce and sesame oil. Whisk to combine.

2. Place a large saute pan over medium-high heat. Cut the baked tofu into 1-inch-by-1/2-inch pieces and add to the marinade. Stir to combine and reserve. Fill a small measuring cup or bowl with cold water and keep by the stovetop.

3. Add the canola oil to the hot pan and swirl to coat. Add the shiitake mushrooms and cook until tender and browned in spots, stirring frequently, about 2 minutes. Add the stir-fry vegetable mix and a large pinch of salt. Cook until crisp tender, 3 to 5 minutes (the cooking time will depend on the size of the vegetables in the mix). If at any

time the pan seems too hot, stir in 1 to 2 tablespoons water. Add the marinated tofu to the vegetables along with 2 tablespoons water. Cook until the tofu is warmed through, 1 to 2 minutes.

4. Transfer the stir-fry to a large platter. Scatter the cashews on top and serve alongside the rice.

Prep: 30 mins

Servings: 6

Ingredients

- 5 medium fennel bulbs, stalks removed
- 1 cup homemade breadcrumbs, or to taste
- ¾ cup finely grated Parmesan cheese
- Black pepper, to taste, freshly ground
- 2 tablespoons olive oil

For the Quick Tomato Sauce:

- 2 tablespoons olive oil
- 1 1/2 pounds ripe plum tomatoes (about 6-8), coarsely chopped
- 1 to 2 cloves garlic, smashed and thinly sliced lengthwise
- 1 small dried red pepper, seeds removed (optional)
- 1/2 teaspoon salt or to taste

- 1 tablespoons, freshly grated Parmesan cheese (optional)

Directions

1. Preheat the oven to 350 degrees F. Halve the fennel bulbs and parboil in salted water for about 10 minutes or until they are just soft and slightly translucent looking. Drain. Cut into quarters. If the bulbs are very large, cut each half into 3 pieces. Set aside.
2. Toss the breadcrumbs and the cheese together in a bowl. Set aside.
3. Bring the Quick Tomato Sauce to a boil over a medium high flame in a wide sauté pan. Lower the heat to medium and simmer until the sauce has thickened, about 10 to 15 minutes. Set aside.
4. Spread a thin layer of tomato sauce on the bottom of a shallow gratin dish. Place the fennel cut sides down on top of the sauce in a tight single layer. Pour the rest of the sauce over them and spread evenly.

5. Sprinkle the fennel with the breadcrumb mixture until you have a generous crust. Drizzle with the olive oil and bake for 30 minutes covered with foil, then 10 minutes uncovered, or until the breadcrumbs are golden.

Prep: 20 mins

Cook: 50 mins

Total: 1 hr 10 mins

Servings: 8

Ingredients

- One 8-ounce bag coleslaw mix
- 4 teaspoons apple cider vinegar
- Kosher salt and freshly ground black pepper
- Two 20-ounce cans jackfruit in brine, rinsed and patted dry
- 2 teaspoon chili powder
- 2 tablespoons vegetable oil
- 3/4 cup barbecue sauce
- 1 to 2 tablespoons light brown sugar, optional
- 8 large potato buns

Directions

1. Combine the coleslaw mix, cider vinegar, 1/2 teaspoon salt and several grinds of black pepper in a medium bowl. Cover with plastic wrap and refrigerate until ready to serve.

2. Combine the jackfruit with the chili powder and 1/2 teaspoon each salt and pepper in a large bowl. Heat 2 tablespoons oil in a large skillet over medium high heat until shimmering. Add the jackfruit and cook, tossing occasionally, until the spices are fragrant 2 to 3 minutes.

3. Add the barbecue sauce to the skillet along with 3 cups water, stir, cover and reduce the heat to low. Cook, stirring occasionally, until tender, 45 to 50 minutes. Uncover the skillet, turn the heat to high and simmer until the color has deepened and the sauce is thick, 4 to 5 minutes. Remove from the heat.

4. Using a potato masher or wooden spoon, smash the jackfruit until it resembles a pulled pork consistency and season to taste with salt, pepper and light brown sugar if you would like it sweeter.

Serve on the potato buns topped with the coleslaw.

Prep: 20 mins

Servings: 4

Ingredients

- 1 teaspoon olive oil
- 1 clove garlic, smashed
- 2 cups packed baby spinach, washed
- 1 tablespoon panko or cornmeal
- 1 whole wheat pizza dough or refrigerated or frozen pizza crust
- ½ cup store bought tomato sauce
- ¾ cup goat cheese
- ½ small onion, halved and thinly sliced
- ½ cup cherry tomatoes or grape tomatoes, halved
- 1 tablespoon olive oil
- Salt and pepper, to taste
- ½ a lemon, zested

Directions

1. Preheat the oven to 500 degrees F. Put 2 baking trays into the oven, or pizza stone if available.

2. In a medium sauté pan, over medium-high heat, add the 1 teaspoon of olive oil and clove of garlic. Cook until the garlic starts to brown and become fragrant. Remove the garlic and add the baby spinach along with 1 tablespoon of water. Let it sit for 1 minute and then stir. Once the spinach has wilted, remove from pan and let it drain. Once cool enough, squeeze out excess liquid.

3. Sprinkle panko or cornmeal onto a large sheet of parchment paper. Roll out the dough onto the parchment paper; press out dough into a 12x8-inch rectangle or to fit your pizza stone. Split into two balls if necessary.

4. Spread the tomato sauce evenly onto the dough. Dot the pizza with the goat cheese and top it with the drained spinach, onions, and grape tomatoes, cut sides up. Drizzle with olive oil and sprinkle with a little salt and pepper.

5. Using the parchment paper, slip the pizza onto the heated baking trays or pizza stone. Bake in the oven on the lowest rack for 10-15 minutes, or until the crust is golden and the cheese looks melted.

6. Using the parchment paper, slip the pizza onto a cutting board. Sprinkle with the lemon zest and cut into slices.

Prep: 10 mins

Cook: 20 miuns

Total: 30 mins

Servings: 6

Ingredients

- 1 small kabocha pumpkin, washed, halved, and seeds scraped out
- 2 tablespoon grape seed or canola oil
- 1 large Spanish onion, thinly sliced
- 8 to 10 cups low-sodium stock or water
- 2 to 3 tablespoons yellow miso paste (miso shiro), or to taste
- Sea salt and black pepper, to taste
- Soy sauce (optional)

Directions

1. With a peeler, take off little patches of skin all over the pumpkin halves until they look polka

dotted. This is purely decorative and can be left out if you don't have time. Cut the halves into a ½-inch dice. Set aside.

2. Heat the oil in a large soup pot over a medium-high flame. When it ripples, add the onion and sauté, stirring until the onion starts to soften and turn transparent. Add the pumpkin cubes, sprinkle with a little sea salt, mix well and cover. Turn the heat down to medium low and sweat the vegetables for about 10 minutes or until the pumpkin has started to soften and the onion is soft. The onion should not brown, so stir the pot occasionally to make sure it doesn't stick.

3. Add enough stock to the pot to cover the vegetables plus 1 inch. Raise the heat and bring to a boil. Cover, turn the heat to low, and simmer until the pumpkin is soft but not mushy, about 10 minutes. Do not overcook! While the soup is cooking, measure the miso into a bowl. Using a small balloon whisk or a fork, gradually whisk in ½ cup of warm stock or cool water until you have a thin-ish, creamy-looking liquid with no lumps.

4. When the pumpkin is tender, add a grind or two
    of black pepper, turn off the heat. Add the miso
    cream little by little, stirring gently to mix. Taste
    as you go until you know how much you like. Miso
    is richly salty, so you do not want too much in the
    soup. Check for seasoning. Serve immediately.

Prep: 20 mins

Cook: 1 hr 25 mins

Total: 1 hr 45 mins

Servings: 12

Ingredients

- Nonstick cooking spray
- 2 cups crispy brown rice cereal
- 1 cup raw pepitas
- 1 cup raw almonds, roughly chopped
- 1/2 cup sweetened dried cherries
- 2/3 cup brown rice syrup
- 2 tablespoons almond butter
- 1/2 teaspoon almond extract
- 1/2 teaspoon flaky sea salt

Directions

1. Preheat an oven to 325 degrees F. Coat an 8-inch square glass baking dish with cooking spray. Line the bottom with a piece of parchment or waxed paper leaving a 4-inch overhang on two opposite sides and spray the paper with cooking spray.

2. Put 1 cup of the rice cereal in a resealable plastic bag and crush to a fine powder with the back of the measuring cup. Combine the remaining 1 cup rice cereal, pepitas, almonds and cherries in a large bowl. Heat the rice syrup and almond butter in a small saucepan until warm and bubbling and remove from heat. Stir in the almond extract and salt, and pour into the nut mixture. Fold with a spatula until it is everything is moistened and well combined. Add the crushed rice cereal and continue to fold until evenly incorporated.

3. Press the mixture very firmly and evenly into the prepared pan using the overhanging pieces of parchment to prevent sticking. Bake until it begins to brown, about 25 minutes. Cool 15 minutes on a wire rack, then press again to compact the mixture. Chill until firm but not completely set, about 45 minutes. Remove the

block by the paper handles and invert onto a cutting board. Gently peel off the paper. Cut the block in half, then cut each half into 6 bars for 12 total. Refrigerate until fully set.

4. Store the bars individually wrapped or layered between sheets of parchment or waxed paper in the refrigerator for up to 2 weeks. The bars will soften up and become chewy as they come to room temperature.

Prep: 20 mins

Cook: 40 mins

Total: 1 hr

Servings: 4

Ingredients

- 12 eggs
- a little olive oil, coconut oil, avocado oil, or grass-fed butter to line the muffin tins
- sea salt and pepper to taste

Veggies:

- Tomato + basil – ¼ cup chopped tomatoes, ¼ cup chopped fresh basil
- Kale + garlic – ½ cup chopped kale, 3 cloves chopped garlic
- Cilantro + green onion – ¼ cup chopped cilantro, ¼ cup green onion.

Directions

1. Preheat oven to 350 degrees F. Lightly grease muffin tins with oil or butter.
2. Chop your choice of veggies
3. Whisk eggs well in a large bowl, add salt and pepper.
4. Stir in veggies
5. Pour into muffin tins.
6. Bake for 20-25 minutes, until eggs are fully cooked through.

Prep: 20 mins

Cook: 25 mins

Total: 45 mins

Servings: 6

Ingredients

- 3 cups small cauliflower florets, chopped
- 2 teaspoons extra-virgin olive oil
- 1 large shallot, minced
- 1 large clove garlic, minced
- Juice of 1 small lemon (about 2 tablespoons)
- 1 tablespoon white or yellow miso paste
- 2 teaspoons spicy mustard
- Kosher salt and freshly ground black pepper
- 1/2 teaspoon ground cayenne pepper
- 1/8 teaspoon ground turmeric
- 3/4 cup plain unsweetened almond or other plant-based milk

- 1/4 cup nutritional yeast flakes

- 2 teaspoons packed brown sugar

- 10 ounces shredded vegan Cheddar (about 2 1/2 cups)

- 1 pound elbow macaroni

Directions

1. Hot sauce, for serving, optional

2. Bring a large pot of water to a boil.

3. Put the cauliflower and 1 cup water in a small saucepan over medium heat. Cover, bring to a simmer and cook until the cauliflower is fully softened, about 20 minutes. Transfer the cooked cauliflower and all the cooking liquid to a food processor and set aside. Wipe out the saucepan.

4. Heat the oil in the saucepan over medium heat. Add the shallot and garlic and cook, stirring, until softened, about 3 minutes. Stir in the lemon juice, miso, mustard, 1 teaspoon salt, 3/4 teaspoon black pepper, cayenne and turmeric until well combined. Gradually whisk in the almond milk,

nutritional yeast and brown sugar and bring just to a simmer. Remove from heat.

5. Process the cauliflower until smooth. With the food processor running, gradually add the warm almond milk mixture and process until extra creamy.

6. Transfer the cauliflower-almond milk mixture to a large saucepan over medium heat, add the vegan Cheddar and stir occasionally until it melts.

7. Meanwhile, add the elbow macaroni to the boiling water and cook according to package directions. Strain, reserving 1 cup of pasta water.

8. Add the pasta to the sauce and stir to combine. Stir in some of the reserved pasta cooking liquid to reach your desired consistency. Add salt to taste. Serve hot with hot sauce on the side if using.

10. Asparagus, Lima Bean & Almond Pasta

Prep: 10 mins

Cook: 10 mins

Total: 20 mins

Servings: 4

Ingredients

- 3 tablespoons almonds, sliced
- 1 tablespoon sea salt, for the pasta water
- 8 ounces whole wheat rotini or penne pasta
- 1 pound green asparagus, trimmed and cut into 1-inch pieces
- 1 cup frozen baby lima beans
- 3 tablespoons olive oil
- 2 cloves garlic, smashed, peeled and thinly sliced
- 1 dried pepper pod, de-seeded (optional)
- 3 tablespoons Italian parsley, chopped
- 1 tablespoon Parmigiano Reggiano cheese, grated (optional)

- Sea salt and black pepper to taste

Directions

1. Toast the sliced almonds in a heavy- wide pan until they are just turning golden. Transfer to a bowl and set aside.

2. Bring salted water to a boil in a large pot. Add pasta to the boiling water and continue to boil for 7 minutes, or 3 minutes less than package instructions. Add the asparagus and frozen lima beans to the boiling pasta and cook for 2 minutes. Reserve 1 cup of pasta water, then drain the pasta and vegetables -- they should be a little undercooked.

3. Meanwhile, in a deep pan or wok, heat olive oil over medium-high heat. Once the oil is hot, add the garlic and chili pepper, if using. Continue cooking until the garlic is light gold, about 3 minutes. Do not let the garlic burn.

4. Add the parsley to the pan and stir-fry for 1 minute. Add ¼ cup of pasta water to the pan and bring to a simmer. Add the almonds, and turn the

heat down to medium. If the pan gets dry, add more pasta water, a little at a time.

5. Add the drained pasta, asparagus, and lima beans to the pan. Stir well, and add in the remaining pasta water, stirring continuously and allowing to reduce. Add the grated cheese and a grind or two of black pepper. Mix well and cook for another minute. Taste for seasonings then serve.

Prep: 15 mins

Servings: 1

Ingredients

- 3 leaves of kale, washed and chopped
- ¼ cup parsley sprigs
- Half of 1 medium apple, cored and cut into chunks
- ⅔ cup fresh or frozen mango, chopped
- 1 teaspoon fresh lemon juice
- ¾ cup cold water, or more if needed
- 2 ice cubes (optional)

Directions

1. Combine all ingredients in a blender and blend until smooth. If you are using fresh mangos, i recommend adding in the ice cubes. Best if served immediately.

Prep: 10 mins

Cook: 20 mins

Total: 30 mins

Servings: 4

Ingredients

- 8 large basil leaves (parsley is good to mix in too)
- 1 clove garlic (or omit and use garlic infused olive oil)
- 1 teaspoon extra-virgin olive oil
- 4 (4 oz) salmon fillets
- 1 pinch salt
- Greens
- 1 clove garlic (or omit and use garlic infused olive oil)
- 2 large bunches Swiss chard
- 1 tablespoon extra-virgin olive oil
- 1 pinch salt

Directions

1. Preheat oven to 375°F.
2. Chop basil and minced garlic (if using).
3. Drizzle baking pan with olive oil or garlic-infused olive oil and place salmon on top.
4. Top salmon with basil, optional garlic, and salt.
5. Bake for about 20 minutes, until salmon flakes easily with a fork.
6. While salmon is baking, prepare greens. Mince garlic (if using) and saute Swiss chard and garlic in olive oil or garlic-infused olive oil and a pinch of salt for 8 minutes or until tender.

Prep: 15 mins

Total: 15 mins

Servings: 2

Ingredients

- ½ ripe Hass avocado
- 2 slices whole-grain toast or good white sourdough toast
- Salt and pepper, to taste
- A drizzle of honey, agave, or olive oil (optional)
- 2 tablespoons sunflower seeds (optional)
- 2 teaspoons ground flaxseed (optional)
- 2 teaspoons chia seed (optional)
- 1 cup arugula, tightly packed

Directions

1. Scoop out the avocado flesh and spread it onto the toast by mashing it with the back of a fork.

Sprinkle salt, pepper, and a drizzle of honey, if using.

2. Add seeds, if using, and top with arugula.

Prep: 15 mins

Servings: 4

Ingredients

- 1 ⅓ cups rolled oats (⅓ cup dry for 1 serving)
- 2 ⅔ cup water (⅔ cup water for ⅓ cup oatmeal)
- Generous pinch sea salt
- 1 tablespoon golden raisins
- 1 tablespoon dried cranberries
- ½ teaspoon cinnamon (optional)
- 2 apples (try tart Granny Smiths or Braeburns)
- 2 tablespoons almonds, sliced, dry toasted
- 2 bananas, thinly sliced
- Milk of your choice, or yogurt to taste

Directions

1. Mix the oats, water, salt, raisins, cranberries, and cinnamon in a pan. Bring to a boil, stir well and

then lower the heat to a low simmer. Cook, covered for about 10 minutes, stirring the oatmeal from time to time so that it doesn't stick.

2. While the oatmeal is cooking, grate the apple using the coarsest bore. When the oatmeal has cooked, stir in the grated apple until it is well mixed. Cover and turn the heat off. Leave the oatmeal for 5 minutes to steam. Serve sprinkled with almonds and sliced bananas, and with milk or yogurt on the side.

Prep: 20 mins

Cook: 6 hrs

Total: 6 hrs 20 mins

Servings: 4

Ingredients

- 2 heads cauliflower, 2-3 pounds in total
- 2 potatoes, medium, peeled, 1-inch chunks
- 4 garlic cloves, peeled
- ¼ cup olive oil
- 4 cups chicken broth, organic, free-range preferred
- 3 cups water
- Salt & freshly ground pepper

When served, add:

- fresh cut herbs, such as thyme, parsley, or chives, if desired

Directions

1. Combine all ingredients, except cheese, in a slow cooker.
2. Cover and cook on low 5 to 6 hours, until vegetables are very tender.
3. Pour into a blender and puree until smooth.
4. Season to taste with salt & pepper and fresh herbs, if desired.

Prep: 15 mins

Servings: 6

Ingredients

- 6 ripe bananas
- 3 tablespoons melted coconut oil
- Freshly grated nutmeg to taste (optional)
- Greek yogurt for serving

Directions

1. Position an oven rack toward the top of the oven. Preheat the oven to 425 degrees. Line a baking tray with parchment paper. Set aside.
2. Pour the melted coconut oil into a shallow bowl or plate.
3. Peel the bananas. Carefully cut them in half lengthwise. Roll them around in the oil until well coated and lay them cut-side down onto the

prepared baking sheet. Brush them with any remaining oil and grate a little nutmeg over them, if using.

4. Bake for 20 minutes on an upper oven rack. Turn the bananas carefully with a spatula — don't break them — and return them to the oven for another 10 minutes or so until they're golden with caramelized edges. Carefully lift them from the tray, and serve warm with a dollop of Greek yogurt.

Prep: 20 mins

Cook: 5 hrs

Total: 5 hrs 20 mins

Servings: 4

Ingredients

- 1 4-pound organic chicken
- salt & pepper
- 3 large garlic cloves
- 6 inches fresh rosemary sprigs
- 1 tablespoon olive oil

Directions

1. Remove neck and giblets from chicken cavity. Liberally salt and pepper chicken inside and out.

2. Place garlic and rosemary inside the cavity. Put chicken in the slow cooker and rub all over with the oil.

3. Cover and cook on low for 5 hours, or until tender and cooked throughout.

4. Remove chicken and cut into serving pieces. Skim fat from the juices. Drizzle juices over the chicken.

Prep: 20 mins

Servings: 6

Ingredients

- 1 small onion, peeled and halved
- 4 whole cloves
- 1 inch slice of lemon peel
- 1 teaspoon whole black peppercorns
- 1 bay leaf
- 1 large carrot, thickly sliced
- 1 stick celery or 2 fennel branches, stripped of their leaves
- 1 teaspoon sea salt, or to taste
- 4 to 6 cups water
- 1 fillet of salmon (about 2 ½ pounds), skin on, bones removed, rinsed and patted dry

Directions

1. Stick the onion halves with the cloves, 2 per half. In a wide sauté pan add the lemon peel, peppercorns, bay leaf, sea salt and all the vegetables, plus enough water to just cover it all. Bring the mixture to a boil over medium-high heat. Cover, turn the heat down to low and simmer until the vegetables begin to soften, about 20 minutes.

2. When the vegetables are cooked, bring the stock back to a gentle boil. Place the salmon skin-side down on top of the vegetables and cover the pan tightly with a lid or foil so that no steam can escape. Turn off the heat.

3. Move the pan to the back of the stove and leave the salmon to steam for 8-10 minutes per inch of thickness, or until it has completely cooled. If you are poaching a whole fillet, check after 15 minutes. Don't open the lid before then -- you will let out all the steam and stop the cooking.

4. When the salmon is ready, gently lift it off the vegetables skin-side down with a plate or cutting

board large enough to hold it in one piece. Take care not to break it. Cover with a second board or a plate big enough to cover it. Carefully flip it over. Remove the skin. Cover with the plate again. Carefully flip it back to right side up. Slide it onto a serving plate, trim, and serve.

Prep: 15 mins

Cook: 55 mins

Total: 1 hr 10 mins

Servings: 4

Ingredients

- 1 medium onion, chopped
- 1 tablespoon olive oil
- 2 bunches collard greens, leaves chopped, stems discarded
- Salt, to taste
- 1 teaspoon smoked paprika
- 2 teaspoons cider or white wine vinegar
- 2 cups chicken or vegetable stock

Directions

1. Heat the olive oil in a medium pot over medium-high heat. Add the onions and cook, stirring occasionally until translucent, about 5-8 minutes.

2. Add the collard greens, sprinkle some salt over them, cover and let steam for 5 minutes.

3. Add the paprika, cook for a minute, then add the cider vinegar, and stock. Cover and cook over low heat for 40 minutes or until very tender.

Prep: 20 mins

Cook: 8 mins

Total: 28 mins

Servings: 4

Ingredients

- 1/2 pounds organic ground organic pork
- 2 tablespoons 100% pure maple syrup
- 1 tablespoon fresh sage
- 1 shallot, finely chopped
- 1 tablespoon Dijon mustard
- 1 teaspoon freshly ground black pepper
- 1 teaspoon kosher salt

Directions

1. Mix all ingredients.
2. Wrap tightly in plastic wrap to keep fresh.

3. Chill in the refrigerator for at least an hour, or
   until ready to cook.
4. When ready to cook, form small patties and cook
   in a skillet over medium heat, turning once, until
   cooked through. About 8 minutes.

Prep: 15 mins

Servings: 2

Ingredients

- 1¼ cup milk or almond milk
- ½ cup whole wheat couscous
- ½ teaspoon cinnamon
- ½ teaspoon ground ginger
- 2 cardamom pods or cloves
- 2 tablespoons chopped almonds
- 2 tablespoons chopped prunes
- 2 tablespoons golden raisins

Directions

1. In a microwave proof bowl, combine the milk with cinnamon, honey, ground ginger, and cardamom. Cover and microwave for 2 minutes, until the milk is very warm and steaming.

2. Remove the bowl from the microwave. Remove the cardamom pods and stir in the couscous. Cover and let sit for 10 minutes, or until the milk has been absorbed. Stir in chopped almonds and dried fruit and enjoy warm.

Prep: 20 mins

Cook: 8 mins

Total: 28 mins

Servings: 4

Ingredients

- 2 cups diced organic apples
- 3 3/4 cups water
- 1/4 cup maple syrup
- 1/2 teaspoon salt
- 2 cups oatmeal
- 6 tablespoons grass-fed butter
- Optional: top with nuts for added nutrition
- Optional: 3/4 teaspoon pumpkin pie spice

Directions

1. Put first four ingredients in a saucepan and bring to a boil.

2. Stir in oatmeal, reduce heat to a simmer, and cook according to the package instructions.

3. While oats cook, cook butter in a small skillet over medium heat until it turns golden brown.

4. Remove butter from heat and add optional pumpkin spice, if using.

5. When oatmeal is done cooking, stir in butter, cover, and let sit for 10 minutes.

6. Serve oatmeal drizzled with remaining spiced brown butter.

Prep: 20 mins

Cook: 45 mins

Total: 1 hr 5 mins

Servings: 6

Ingredients

- 1 large bunch young collard greens or 2 small ones, leaves stripped from the hard stems and washed
- 1 to 2 tablespoons olive oil
- 1 sprig plus 1 teaspoon of fresh rosemary, leaves stripped and chopped
- 1 medium onion, finely diced
- 1 large carrot, cut into a small dice
- 1 medium Yukon Gold potato or other waxy potato, cut into a small dice
- 1 clove garlic, chopped

- 2 cups cooked baby lima or other white beans (cannellini or Great Northern), plus their broth or 1 (14-ounce) can, drained and rinsed well, plus ½ cup fresh water
- 2¼ quarts (9 cups) low-sodium vegetable or chicken stock, or water
- 1 tablespoon chopped flat-leaf parsley

Directions

1. Pull the leaves from their stems. Cut the leaves into bite-sized pieces. Set aside.
2. In a large Dutch oven, heat the oil over a medium-high flame until it starts to ripple. Add the rosemary. Let it sizzle for a moment, then add the onion, carrot, and potato. Mix well.
3. Turn the heat down to medium-low. Cover and sweat the vegetables for 8-10 minutes or until they are soft and the onion is slightly golden. Stir every so often to prevent sticking or burning.
4. Turn the heat up to medium high. Add the chopped garlic. Stir and cook for another 2

minutes until you start to smell its aroma. Add the collard greens and stir-fry until they start to wilt and soften.

5. Add the stock and beans, plus their liquid if home-cooked. The beans and vegetables should be well covered with liquid but not drowned. Add a little extra water if needed. Bring the soup to a boil. Partially cover and turn the heat down to low. Simmer, stirring from time to time, for 20-25 minutes or until the greens are very tender.

6. Adjust seasoning, then cook 5 minutes more. Mash some of the beans against the sides of the pan to thicken the soup slightly. Stir in the chopped parsley and remaining rosemary. Cook 1 minute, then turn off the heat. Let the soup sit, covered, for 5 minutes. Serve drizzled with a little olive oil, if desired.

Prep: 15 mins

Total: 15 mins

Servings: 14

Ingredients

- ½ cup plus 2 tablespoons smooth all natural peanut butter
- ¼ cup white miso paste
- 1 tablespoon honey
- 1 tablespoon water

Directions

1. In a medium bowl, beat the peanut butter, miso paste, honey, and water together until they are completely blended.
2. If you want a softer or a runnier consistency, gradually add more water a teaspoon at a time until it is how you want it.

Prep: 15 mins

Servings: 4

Ingredients

- 6 cups homemade Chicken Stock or Basic Vegetable Stock
- 16 oz of egg nest pasta
- 4 cups of baby spinach
- Parmesan cheese (optional)

Directions

1. Bring the broth to a boil. Break the pasta into the broth and cook until just tender. Break up the pasta with a kitchen knife if you want the noodles shorter.
2. Stir in the spinach, and cook for 2 more minutes. Serve with a little Parmesan cheese, if desired.

Prep: 5 mins

Cook: 30 mins

Total: 35 mins

Servings: 4

Ingredients

- 3 bunches of Lacinato kale, leaves stripped
- 6 cloves of garlic, smashed and skinned
- 1 teaspoon sea salt, or to taste
- ¼ cup extra virgin olive oil
- Freshly grated nutmeg, to taste

Directions

1. Put the kale and the whole garlic cloves into a large non-reactive pan with a lid. Add salt and just enough water to cover. Bring to a boil, then cover and simmer until the leaves are tender,

about 15 – 20 minutes. Reserve a cup of the cooking water then drain.

2. Blend the cooked kale and garlic into a blender with olive oil, nutmeg, and ¼ cup of the reserved broth. Add more of the reserved water, a little at a time, if the sauce seems too stiff. The sauce should be very thick but pourable. Adjust seasoning and serve tossed with a short whole wheat pasta and freshly grated parmesan.

Prep: 10 mins

Cook: 10 mins

Total: 20 mins

Servings: 4

Ingredients

- ⅔ cup water
- Salt, to taste
- 1 dark green scallion stem
- 1 piece of lemon peel, about 2 inches
- ¾ cup fresh or frozen peas
- ¾ cup chopped baby spinach
- 1 cup regular or whole-wheat couscous
- Black pepper, to taste
- 2 tablespoons chopped scallions, white and light green parts only
- 4 Poached Eggs

Directions

1. In a medium stockpot, add the water, salt, scallion stem, and lemon peel, and bring to a boil.
2. Add the peas and baby spinach and continue to boil for 2 minutes. Turn off the heat, then stir in the couscous. Cover and let sit for 5 minutes.
3. Add the black pepper and chopped scallions, if using, and fluff the couscous with a fork. Taste for seasoning. Serve topped with a poached egg.

Prep: 15 mins

Total: 15 mins

Servings: 1

Ingredients

- ¼ cup rolled oats
- ¼ cup water
- 1 cup milk of your choice
- 1 large ripe banana, peeled and cut into thirds
- 1 to 2 tablespoons unsweetened and unsalted peanut butter, or almond butter
- 2 teaspoons honey, or to taste
- ¼ to ½ teaspoon freshly ground nutmeg
- 2 ice cubes(optional)

Directions

1. In a microwave-safe bowl, combine the oats and water and microwave on high for 1 minute.

Alternatively, cook the oats in a small saucepan until the water has been absorbed. Set aside and let cool.

2. In a blender, combine the oatmeal, milk, banana, peanut butter, honey, nutmeg, and ice cubes, if using. Blend until smooth. Best if served right away.

Prep: 20 mins

Cook: 1 hr

Total: 1 hr 20 mins

Servings: 4

Ingredients

- 2 tablespoons olive oil
- 1 small onion, chopped
- 3 bay leaves
- Pinch of cayenne
- ¼ teaspoon brown sugar
- 2 pounds tomatoes, diced or 1 (28-ounce) can of chopped tomatoes
- 6 to 8 cloves of garlic, smashed and peeled
- 1 quart low-sodium stock or water
- ¼ cups pearl barley
- Parmesan rind (optional)
- Sea salt, to taste

- Fresh basil

Directions

1. Heat the oil over medium-high heat in a wide, heavy-bottomed pan. Add the onion and cook for a minute. Turn the heat to medium, add the bay leaves and sweat the onion until it starts to soften, about 8 minutes. It shouldn't color, so stir from time to time to prevent it sticking and burning.

2. Turn the heat up to medium-high. Add the cayenne pepper, sugar and cook for a minute, then add the tomatoes and garlic. Cook, stirring until the tomatoes take on an orangey hue and have reduced a little.

3. Add the pearl barley, Parmesan rind, if using, and the stock, plus salt to taste. Bring to a simmer, lower the heat and cover. Cook until the barley is tender enough to smash with a spoon against the side of the pan, about 40 minutes. If substituting Arborio rice, it will take about half the amount of time to cook.

4. Let the soup sit for a few minutes. Remove the bay leaves and blend thoroughly, in batches, using either a wand blender or a freestanding one. Return to the pot, check the seasoning and add a grind or two of black pepper. Serve as is or with a few torn basil leaves or a little pesto stirred into it.

Prep: 15 mins

Cook: 30 mins

Total: 45 mins

Servings: 6

Ingredients

- 2 tablespoons extra-virgin olive oil
- 1 cup chopped onion (from about 1/2 medium onion)
- Kosher salt
- 1/2 cup chopped celery (from about 1 medium stalk)
- 1 clove garlic, smashed
- Freshly ground black pepper
- 2 medium Yukon gold potatoes, peeled and diced (about 3/4 pound)
- 4 cups broccoli florets
- 1/2 cup unsweetened soy milk

- 1/4 cup nutritional yeast
- 1/4 teaspoon freshly grated nutmeg

Directions

1. Heat the oil in a large saucepan over medium heat. Add the onions and 1/2 teaspoon salt and cook until light brown, about 7 minutes. Add the celery, garlic and 1/4 teaspoon pepper and cook for 5 minutes. Add the potatoes, 4 cups water and 1/2 teaspoon salt, raise the heat to high and bring to a boil. Return the heat to medium, cover and cook until the potatoes are tender, about 15 minutes. Add the broccoli, cover and cook until the broccoli is bright green, about 5 minutes.

2. Transfer the soup to a blender; add the soy milk and puree until smooth, leaving the filler cap slightly open to let steam escape (or puree the soup in the pot with an immersion blender). Return the soup to the saucepan and bring to a simmer; stir in the nutritional yeast and nutmeg.

Add water if needed to adjust consistency and add salt and pepper to taste.

www.ingramcontent.com/pod-product-compliance
Lightning Source LLC
Chambersburg PA
CBHW071949120726
48001CB00005B/2107